11/4/97

W9-CJX-532

WITHDRAWN

Blood Circulation

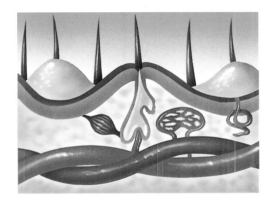

Andres Llamas Ruiz
Illustrations by Luis Rizo

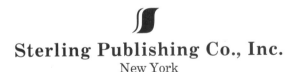

Sterling Publishing Co., Inc.
New York

Illustrations by Luis Rizo
Text by Andres Llamas Ruiz
Translated by Natalia Tizón

Library of Congress Cataloging-in-Publication Data

Llamas Ruiz, Andrés.
   [Circulación de la sangre. English]
   Blood circulation / Andres Llamas Ruiz.
         p.   cm. — (Cycles of life)
   Includes index.
   Summary: Explains how blood circulates in our bodies and the specific roles that the heart, lungs, and blood vessels play.
   ISBN 0-8069-9331-6
   1. Blood—Circulation—Juvenile literature.   [1. Blood—Circulation.   2. Circulatory system.]   I. Title.   II. Series: Llamas Ruiz, Andrés.   Secuencias de la naturaleza.   English.
   QP103.L5613   1996
   612.1—dc20   96–9201
                                                                              CIP
                                                                              AC

1   3   5   7   9   10   8   6   4   2

Published by Sterling Publishing Company, Inc.
387 Park Avenue South, New York, N.Y. 10016
Originally published in Spain by Ediciones Estes
©1996 by Ediciones Estes, S.A. ©1996 by Ediciones Lema, S.L.
English version and translation © 1996 by Sterling Publishing Company, Inc.
Distributed in Canada by Sterling Publishing
% Canadian Manda Group, One Atlantic Avenue, Suite 105
Toronto, Ontario, Canada M6K 3E7
Distributed in Great Britain and Europe by Cassell PLC
Wellington House, 125 Strand, London WC2R 0BB, England
Distributed in Australia by Capricorn Link (Australia) Pty Ltd.
P.O. Box 6651, Baulkham Hills, Business Centre, NSW 2153, Australia
Printed and Bound in Spain

Sterling ISBN 0-8069-9331-6

Table of Contents

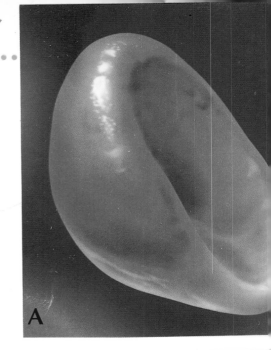

A

Blood travels through a very complex network of arteries, veins, and capillaries.

Blood performs two very important functions: it transports oxygen and nutrients to all the cells throughout the organism and it collects waste from the cells. Waste products are then expelled through the kidneys, skin, and lungs.

How much blood travels through this complex system? In adults, over 5 quarts (5 liters) of blood are constantly pumped by the heart.

If you examine blood through a microscope, you will see a liquid called "plasma," in which different kinds of cells or "corpuscles" float.

The most important blood cells are composed of three types: red cells (erythrocytes), white cells (leukocytes), and platelets (thrombocytes).

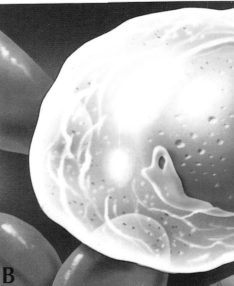

B

1

Plasma is the liquid component of blood.

1. Substances such as proteins, sugar, minerals, hormones, and many others travel in plasma.

2. Approximately 52% of blood is made up of plasma, while 46% is made up of platelets, and red and white blood cells.

3. Red cells cannot move on their own; they are carried through the body by the bloodstream.

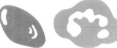

You can see here the three main types of blood cells:
A. *Red cells (erythro-cytes)*
B. *White cells (leuko-cytes)*
C. *Platelets (thrombo-cytes)*

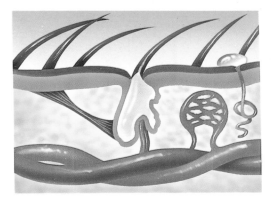

Cold. Contraction of the capillaries

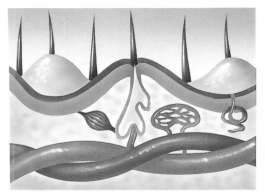

Heat. Dilation of the capillaries

Blood also acts as a heating mecha-nism. It helps to keep the body temperature constant by carrying heat from one part of the body to another.

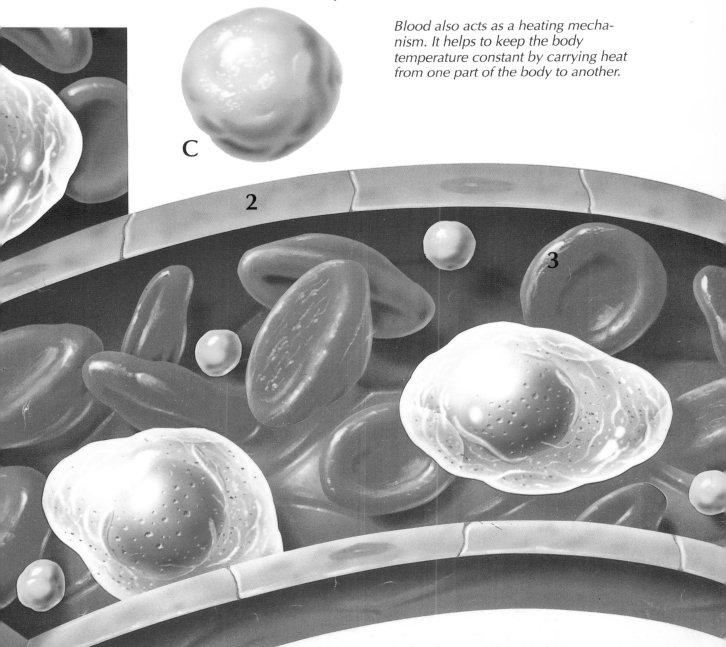

C

2

3

Blood always starts and ends its journey at the heart.

A stream of blood travels among the organs and cells of the human body in a voyage that covers approximately 10 miles every hour.

Fresh, oxygenated blood starts the trip to the body's tissues after passing through the left side of the heart. It makes one complete trip through the body every 20 seconds. This means it repeats the process 4,320 times per day.

The blood circulation in humans is "complete and double." It is "double" because there are two circulation systems: the systematic and the pulmonary. The systematic travels through the body and brings food and oxygen to the cells. Pulmonary circulation forces blood from the heart to the lungs, where there is an exchange of gases during which the blood is purified.

The circulation is "complete" because the blood of the systematic and the blood of the pulmonary circulation systems do not mix.

1

1. Blood full of oxygen leaves the left ventricle through the aorta artery.

2. Then the blood enters the three smaller arteries that carry it to the organs of the upper body.

3. The aorta branches out to form the diverse arteries that reach the body's organs. In each organ or in each part of the body, arteries branch out and form the capillary network that carries nutrients and energy to all cells.

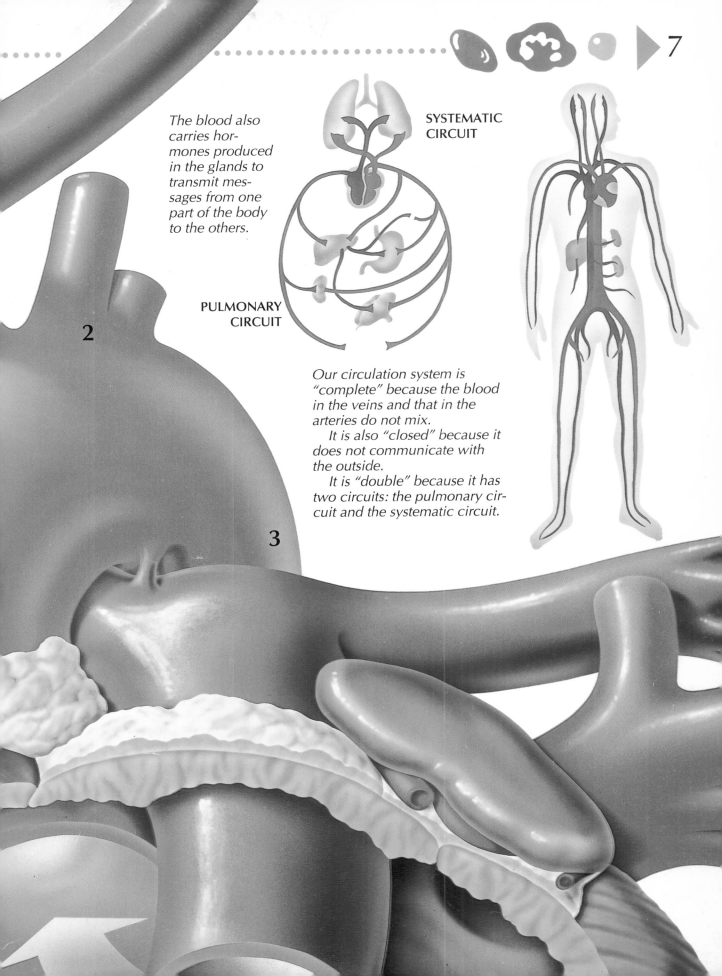

The blood also carries hormones produced in the glands to transmit messages from one part of the body to the others.

SYSTEMATIC CIRCUIT

PULMONARY CIRCUIT

2

3

Our circulation system is "complete" because the blood in the veins and that in the arteries do not mix.

It is also "closed" because it does not communicate with the outside.

It is "double" because it has two circuits: the pulmonary circuit and the systematic circuit.

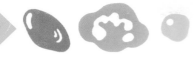

Oxygenated arterial blood flows out of the heart to the body's tissues.

Arteries are the blood vessels through which blood is pumped out of the heart, traveling to the body's tissues and organs. For the blood to reach all parts of the body, the heart has to pump very hard. This means that blood travels through the veins "by pressure." To support this pressure, the interior walls of the arteries are made of an elastic tissue. The aorta—the human body's largest artery—can withstand the rush of blood pumping out of the heart at seventy times per minute.

Healthy, young arteries are elastic tubes with smooth walls through which blood flows rapidly with little friction. However, old and calcified arteries (called sclerotic) have rough, rigid, fragile walls, which make it difficult for the blood to circulate. In these veins, blood moves slowly, which strains the heart and can lead to the formation of clots. If one of the vessels clogs, it can cause very serious damage.

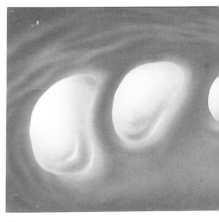

A

Because of age or disease, the interior of the arteries changes.
A. *Healthy artery with smooth, elastic walls.*
B. *Sick, sclerotic artery with rough walls and a clot. In this kind of artery, blood has trouble circulating properly, which strains the heart. This condition is sometimes called "hardening of the arteries."*

As you can see, most parts of the body have a very complete and complex network of arteries. That is how they ensure that vital organs receive enough oxygen and nutrients.

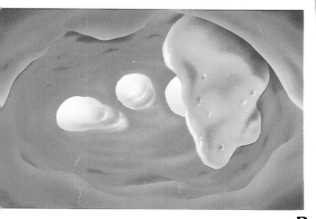

B

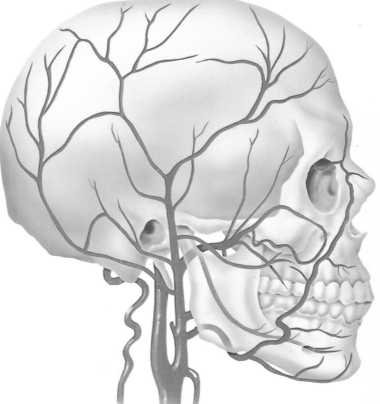

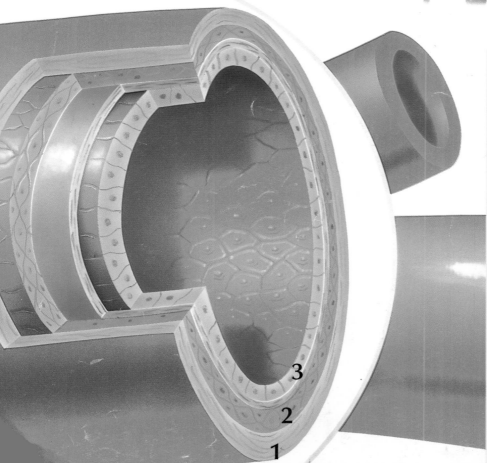

3

2

1

Two arteries extend from the heart. The aorta branches out through the rest of the body in the systematic circulation network. The pulmonary artery pumps blood to the lungs in the pulmonary circulation system.

Regardless of their size and function, all arteries are made of three layers of cells:

1. Tunica adventitia (exterior layer): an external layer of connective tissue.

2. Tunica media (center layer): made of smooth, muscular fiber, powerful and elastic, which allows the artery to vary in diameter, depending on the needs of the body.

3. Tunica intima (interior layer): made of flattened cells, which allows the blood to flow easily within the artery.

Oxygen travels in disk-shaped red cells, which have no nucleus.

Red blood cells are very abundant, making up 46% of the volume of blood. However, they are so small that if we put five hundred of them one on top of the other, they would be less than 1 inch (1 cm) in height.

The ability to transport oxygen and carbon dioxide depends on the presence of a very special molecule called hemoglobin that is inside the red cell. Hemoglobin is a protein formed by four "hemo" groups (containing iron) to which oxygen attaches in order to be transported.

The average life span of a red cell is 120 days. It is "born" from a stem cell in the red bone marrow of the long bones. This process is constant. As a red cell ages, it becomes deformed and fragile. Old cells accumulate in the spleen, where they are destroyed or "die" at a rate of two million every second. However, before dying, each of them has traveled more than 75,000 times between the lungs and the other tissues.

This is what a hemoglobin molecule looks like. It is a pigment that gives the typical red color to blood and transports oxygen from the lungs to the cells.

1. Red bone marrow is found at the ends of long bones. In it are the stem cells that will create the blood cells.

2. Red cells do not have a nucleus; they are very small. There are five million of them in each cubic millimeter of blood! White cells have both nucleus and granules. Platelets are formed when a stem cell becomes a large cell that divides into smaller ones.

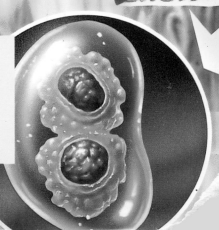

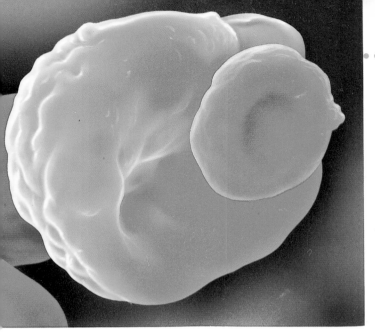

You can see how a leukocyte that is in charge of cleaning catches an old erythrocyte. The leukocyte swallows and digests the old cell. This is how many red cells are retired from "active service."

To form a new erythrocyte, the cell has to get rid of the nucleus from its inside. It then adopts the shape of a disk and flows into the bloodstream.

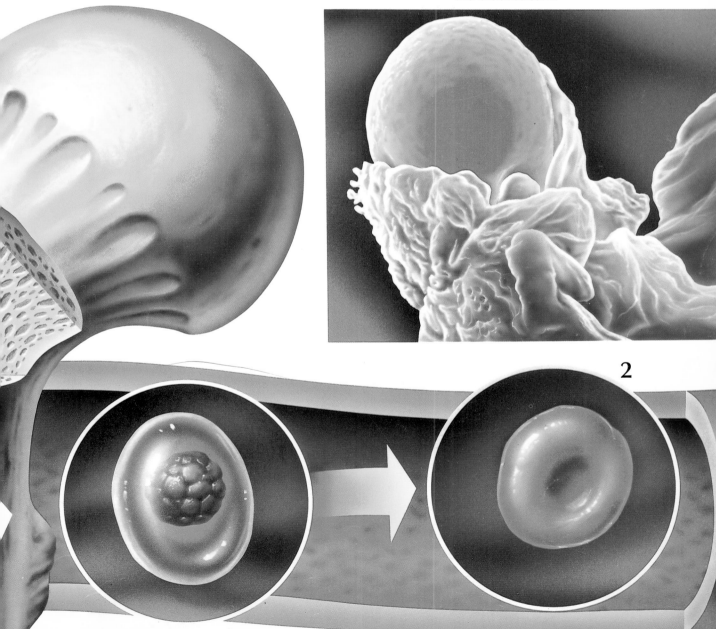

2

White cells or leukocytes are in charge of defense.

Leukocytes are bigger than red cells; however, there are fewer of them: There are only 5,000 to 10,000 per cubic millimeter of blood. These cells act as the body's "police." They travel in the bloodstream, watching for and devouring bacteria, viruses, and other microscopic invaders. When there is an infection and a strange agent enters the body, white cells destroy it. Unlike red cells, white cells move on their own by using false legs called pseudopodia. They also move out of the blood vessels to get to an area where there is an invasion of enemy bacteria.

Leukocytes have a very short life span, living just a few days. When they die fighting bacteria, they form pus, which consists of dead leukocytes, dead and live bacteria, and cell waste swimming in lymph.

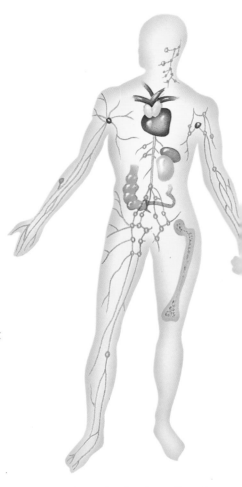

When the body suffers from a infectious episode, such as appendicitis, the number of leukocytes increases in a defensive reaction in order to better fight off the infection. There are several organs throughout the body that produce white cells.

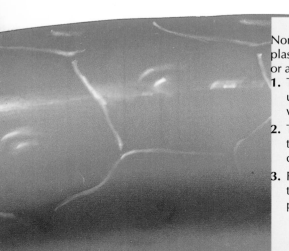

Normally, white cells swim in plasma until they detect bacteria or a foreign body.
1. The leukocyte approaches until it comes into contact with the invader.
2. Then it wraps itself around the invader, forcing it into the cytoplasm of the white cell.
3. Finally, the leukocyte digests the invading agent in a process called phagocytosis.

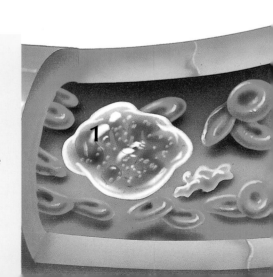

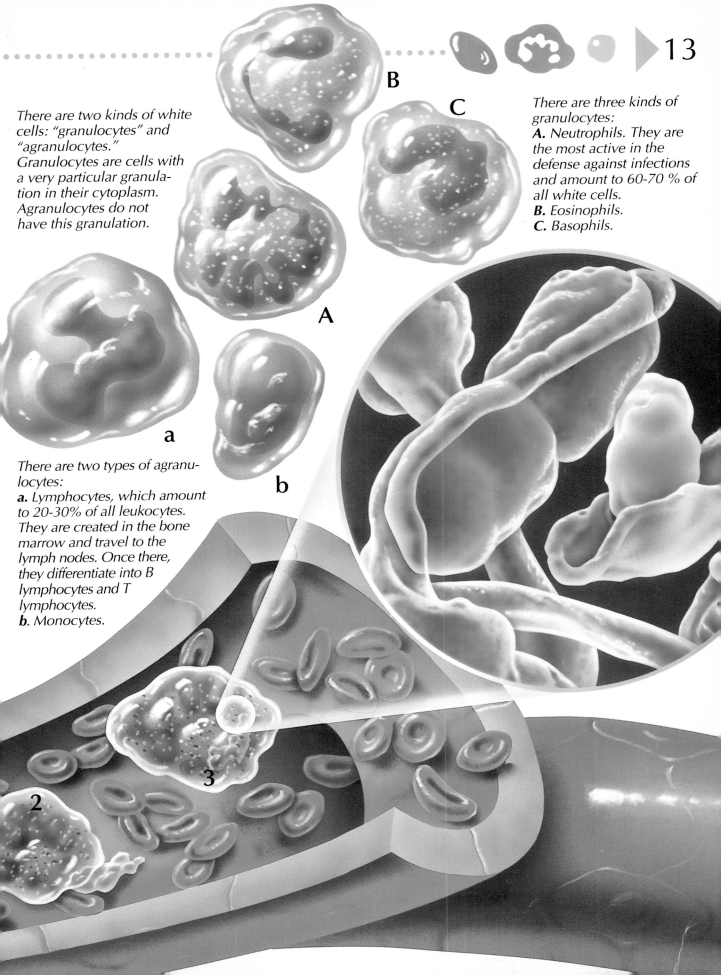

There are two kinds of white cells: "granulocytes" and "agranulocytes." Granulocytes are cells with a very particular granulation in their cytoplasm. Agranulocytes do not have this granulation.

There are three kinds of granulocytes:
A. Neutrophils. They are the most active in the defense against infections and amount to 60-70 % of all white cells.
B. Eosinophils.
C. Basophils.

There are two types of agranulocytes:
a. Lymphocytes, which amount to 20-30% of all leukocytes. They are created in the bone marrow and travel to the lymph nodes. Once there, they differentiate into B lymphocytes and T lymphocytes.
b. Monocytes.

Arteries branch out and reduce in diameter until they become arterial capillaries.

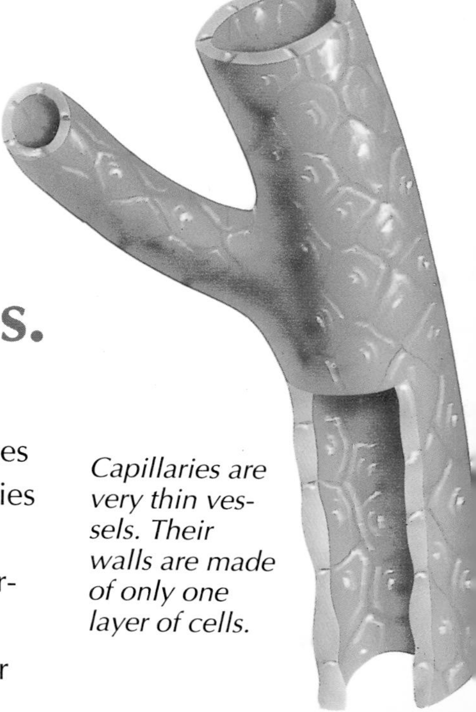

In this way, the exchange of substances and gases becomes easier. In addition to transporting oxygen, blood also carries ions, such as sodium, chlorine, potassium, vitamins, fats, sugar, proteins, mineral salts—all of which are very important for the life of all cells in the body.

Capillaries are very thin vessels with a diameter similar to that of a hair. Their walls only have one layer of cells. In fact, they are so narrow that red cells have to bend and twist, traveling one by one, to be able to circulate through them!

Most tissues have a network of capillaries so complete and dense that there is only a tiny fraction of an inch to the nearest source of blood.

After an exchange with a tissue's cells, arterial capillaries become vein capillaries, which help start the blood's return to the heart.

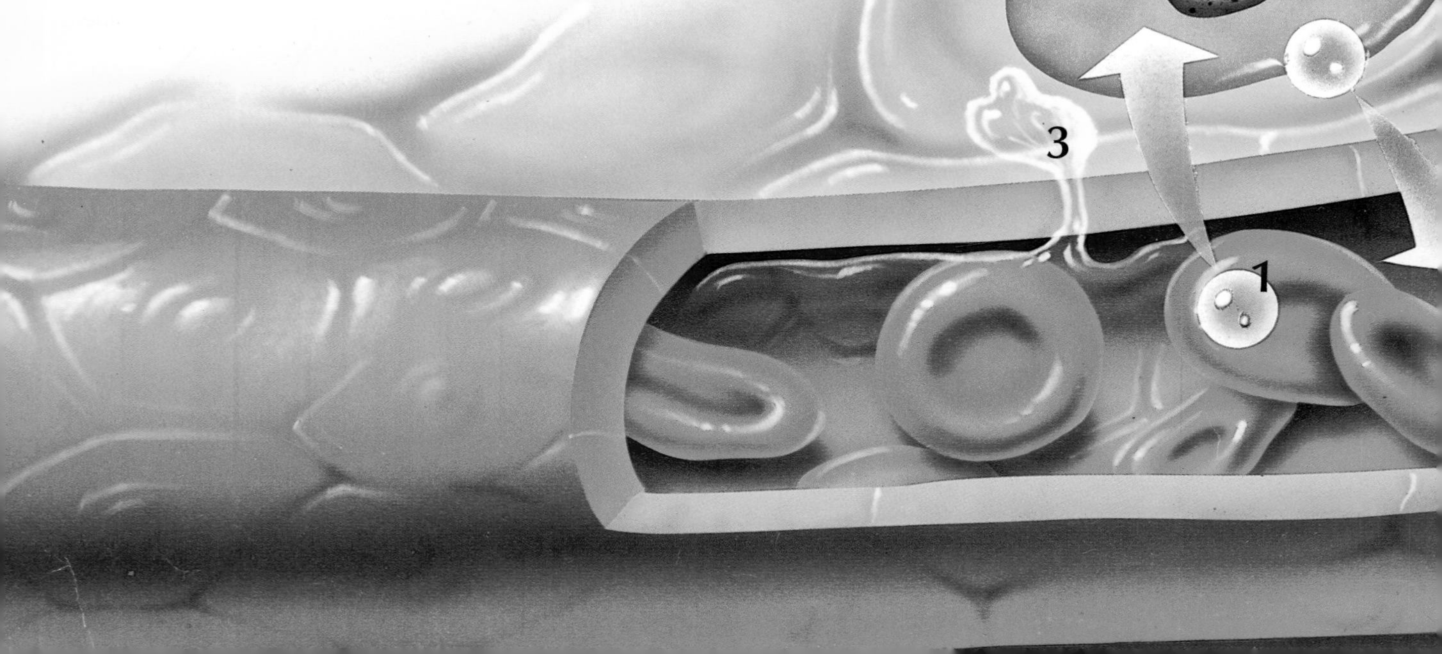

Capillaries are very thin vessels. Their walls are made of only one layer of cells.

3

1

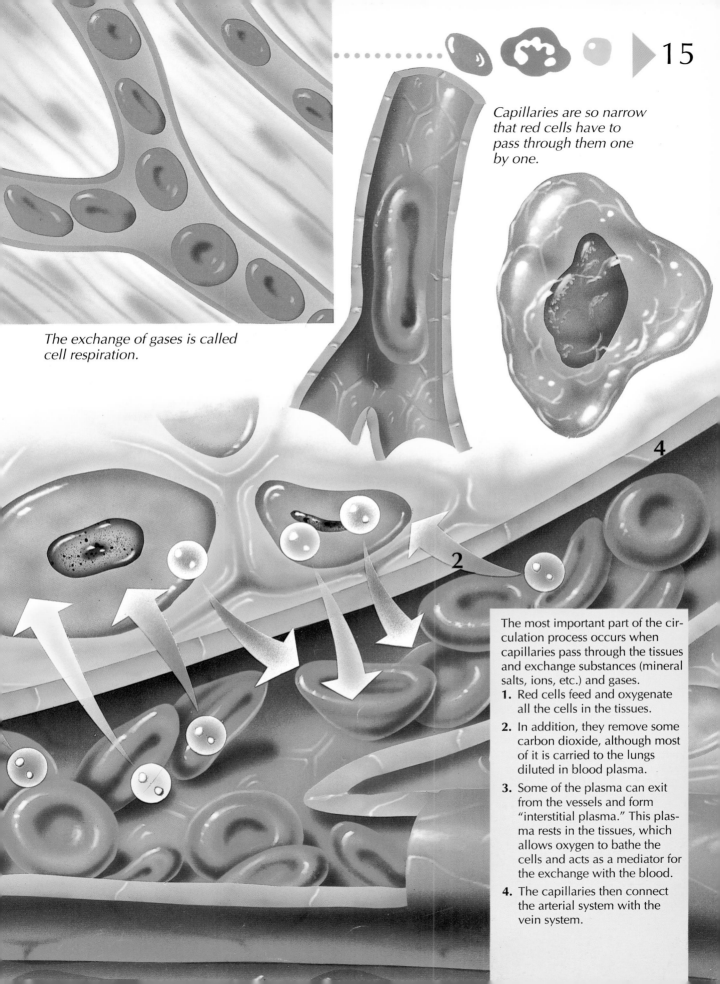

Capillaries are so narrow that red cells have to pass through them one by one.

The exchange of gases is called cell respiration.

4

2

The most important part of the circulation process occurs when capillaries pass through the tissues and exchange substances (mineral salts, ions, etc.) and gases.

1. Red cells feed and oxygenate all the cells in the tissues.

2. In addition, they remove some carbon dioxide, although most of it is carried to the lungs diluted in blood plasma.

3. Some of the plasma can exit from the vessels and form "interstitial plasma." This plasma rests in the tissues, which allows oxygen to bathe the cells and acts as a mediator for the exchange with the blood.

4. The capillaries then connect the arterial system with the vein system.

There are ways of preventing blood loss when a vessel is damaged.

Platelets (thrombocytes) are responsible for blood coagulation (clotting). Small and flat, with no nucleus, there are 200,000 to 350,000 of them per cubic millimeter of blood. Technically, they are not actually cells but small pieces of the cytoplasm from very large cells called megacariocytes. Platelets are formed in the bone marrow. They have a short life span, living for only seven days.

Many processes occur during coagulation. Vessel constriction—the narrowing of a damaged blood vessel—may be enough to close the hole of the wound in the thinnest of the vessels. If, however, a wound affects a medium-size vessel, platelets will accumulate there like tiny bricks to close off a tear or hole.

If a wound is very big, platelets need to form a support structure that acts like cement connecting the bricks of a wall. This structure, called fibrin, forms a lid-like type of net called a "clot" where red cells are trapped and, thus, prevent blood from escaping.

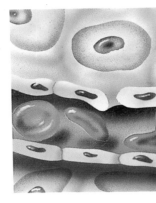

The intervention of platelets is not always necessary. For example, if a very thin capillary is wounded, vessel constriction will occur, and the walls of the vessel will contract until the wound is closed.

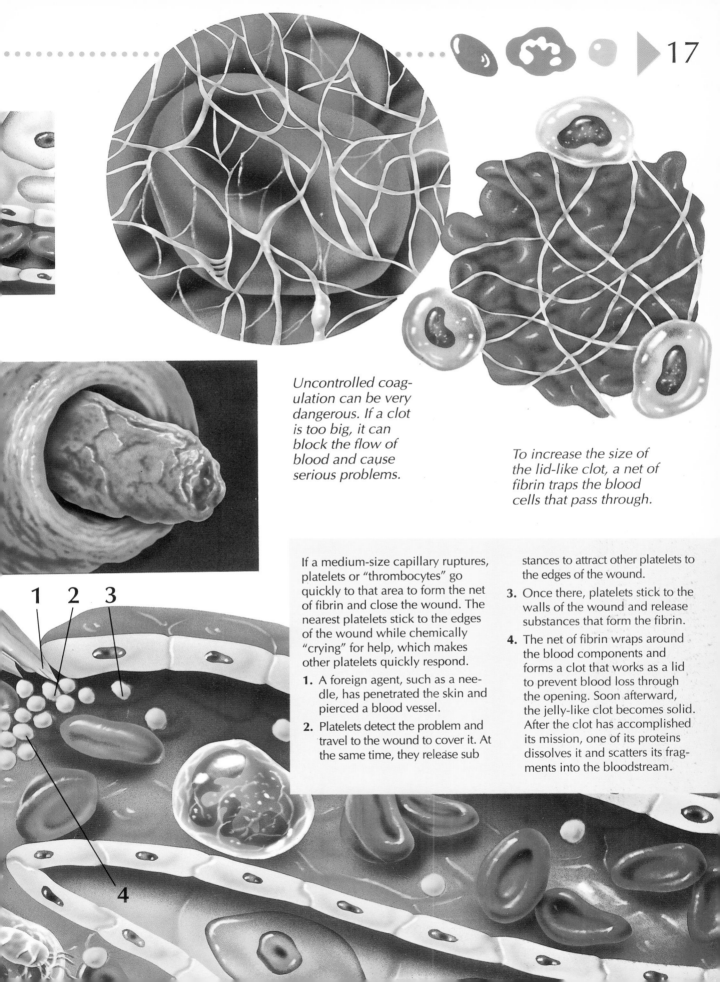

Uncontrolled coag-ulation can be very dangerous. If a clot is too big, it can block the flow of blood and cause serious problems.

To increase the size of the lid-like clot, a net of fibrin traps the blood cells that pass through.

If a medium-size capillary ruptures, platelets or "thrombocytes" go quickly to that area to form the net of fibrin and close the wound. The nearest platelets stick to the edges of the wound while chemically "crying" for help, which makes other platelets quickly respond.

1. A foreign agent, such as a nee-dle, has penetrated the skin and pierced a blood vessel.

2. Platelets detect the problem and travel to the wound to cover it. At the same time, they release sub

stances to attract other platelets to the edges of the wound.

3. Once there, platelets stick to the walls of the wound and release substances that form the fibrin.

4. The net of fibrin wraps around the blood components and forms a clot that works as a lid to prevent blood loss through the opening. Soon afterward, the jelly-like clot becomes solid. After the clot has accomplished its mission, one of its proteins dissolves it and scatters its frag-ments into the bloodstream.

1   2   3

4

T hen the vein blood picks up the cell waste.

After passing through the capillary network, erythrocytes arrive at an area where capillaries connect to form veins (kidney veins, hepatic veins). The large vena cava goes to the right auricle of the heart. All these veins are responsible for carrying erythrocytes back to the heart.

Veins are less elastic than arteries. Inside the larger veins there is an interesting system of "anti-reversal" valves, which prevent the blood from flowing backward.

Like the arteries, veins have three layers of tissue. However, the center tunica is thinner. This explains why veins are softer and more fragile, as well as less elastic.

The only veins that carry "arterial" blood to the heart are the pulmonary veins, since they come from the lungs and carry oxygenated blood. The rest of the veins run parallel to the arteries and carry vein blood.

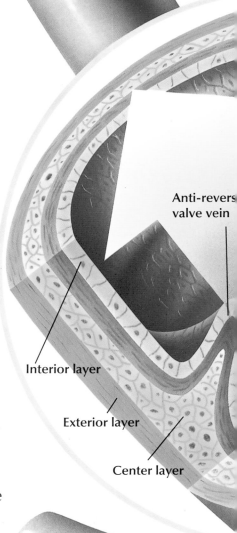

Anti-reversal valve vein

Interior layer

Exterior layer

Center layer

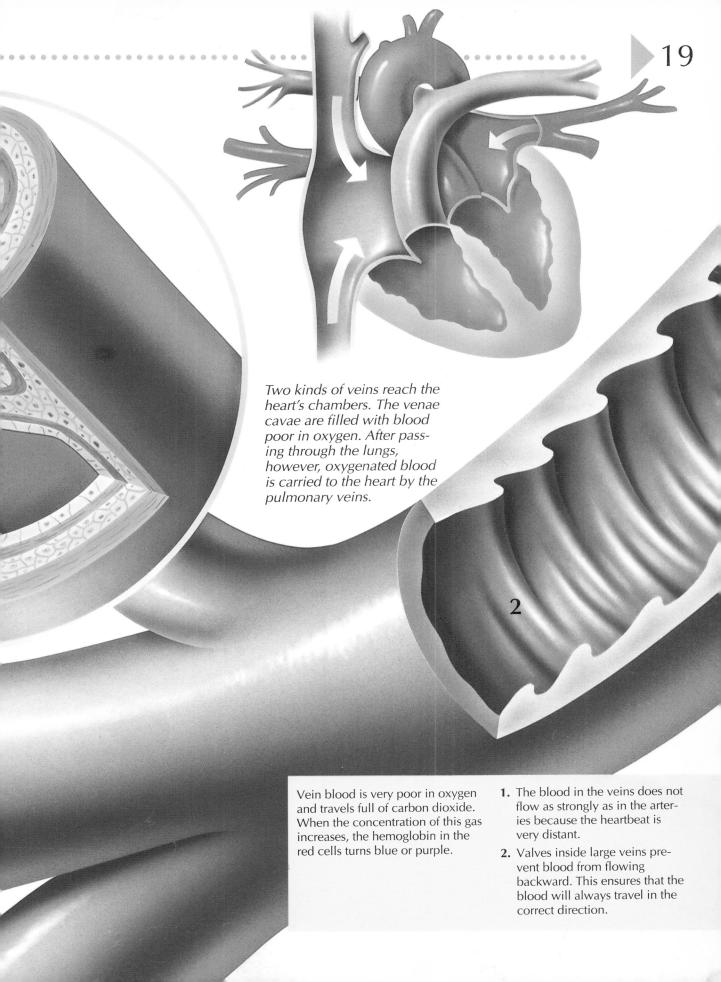

Two kinds of veins reach the heart's chambers. The venae cavae are filled with blood poor in oxygen. After passing through the lungs, however, oxygenated blood is carried to the heart by the pulmonary veins.

2

Vein blood is very poor in oxygen and travels full of carbon dioxide. When the concentration of this gas increases, the hemoglobin in the red cells turns blue or purple.

1. The blood in the veins does not flow as strongly as in the arteries because the heartbeat is very distant.

2. Valves inside large veins prevent blood from flowing backward. This ensures that the blood will always travel in the correct direction.

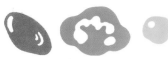

Vein blood returns to the heart, which works as a pump.

The heart of an adult is the size of a fist and weighs between 10.5 and 17.5 ounces (300 and 500 grams). Hollow inside, it is divided in half by a central wall. The left side of the heart is the more muscular side, since it is in charge of pumping blood through the body. The right side pumps blood to the lungs, where it will be oxygenated. The central wall prevents oxygenated and vein blood from mixing.

In each half of the heart there are two cavities. The upper ones are auricles and the lower ones are ventricles. Between both of these is a hole surrounded by tendon-like rings that let the blood pass through in only one direction. These are the cardiac valves and they are responsible for circulating blood in the correct direction—always from the auricles to the ventricles.

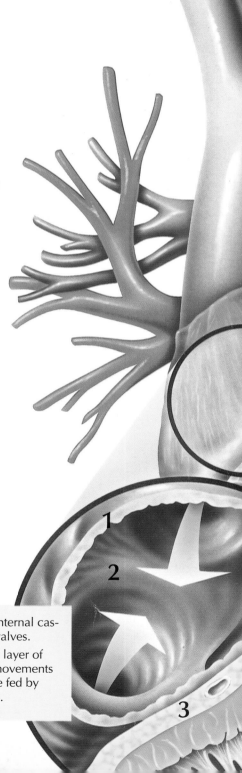

The heart is made up of three layers: pericardium, myocardium, and endocardium.
1. The pericardium is the exterior skin that protects the heart and fixes it to the neighboring structures.
2. The endocardium is an elastic tissue covering the inside of the internal casing that forms the cardiac valves.
3. The myocardium forms the layer of muscle where the heart's movements originate; these muscles are fed by cardiac or coronary vessels.

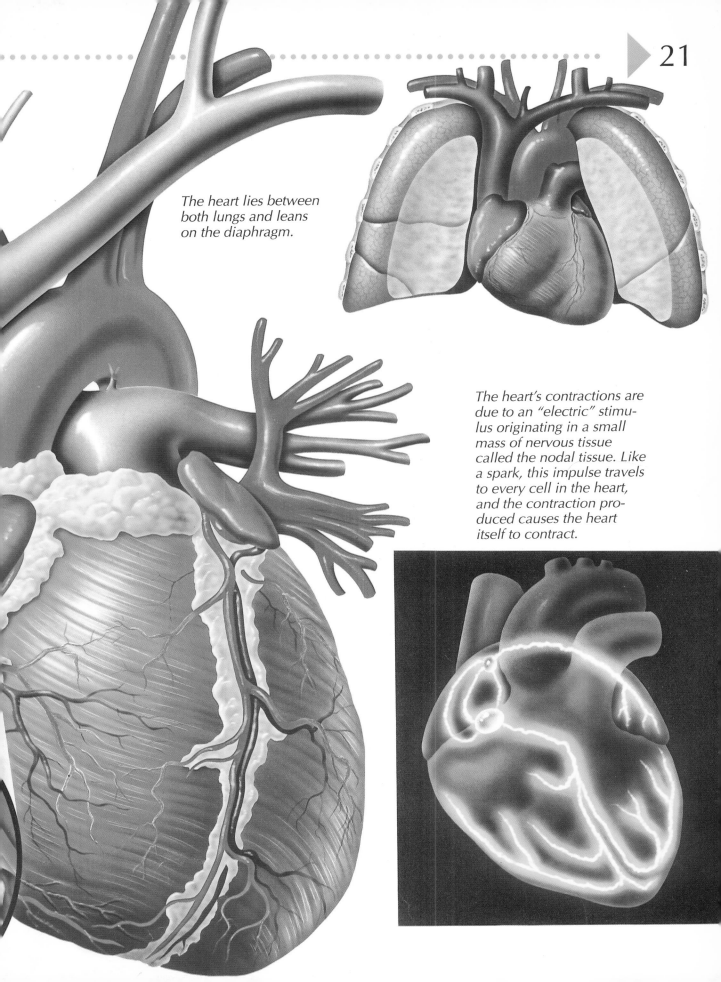

The heart lies between both lungs and leans on the diaphragm.

The heart's contractions are due to an "electric" stimulus originating in a small mass of nervous tissue called the nodal tissue. Like a spark, this impulse travels to every cell in the heart, and the contraction produced causes the heart itself to contract.

Heartbeat is caused by the contraction of the ventricles.

The heart constantly and alternatively performs two kinds of movement: systole and diastole. Systole is a contraction movement that expels blood from the heart. Diastole is a dilation movement in which the heart becomes full of the blood carried to the auricle by the vena cava and pulmonary veins. Out of the right ventricle comes the pulmonary artery that carries vein blood to the lung for oxygenation. Out of the left ventricle comes the aorta, which branches out through the body.

The "pulse" is the most simple way "to feel" the heartbeat. You can feel your own pulse by placing your index finger on a superficial artery like the one on your wrist or on the carotid artery on your neck. The heart beats about seventy times per minute; the heart of a 75-year-old person has beat more than 2,500 million times!

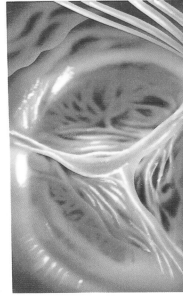

A

Cardiac valves allow the blood to pass in only one direction from the auricles to the ventricles. Here, you can see one of these valves (the tricuspid valve) closed (A) and opened (B).

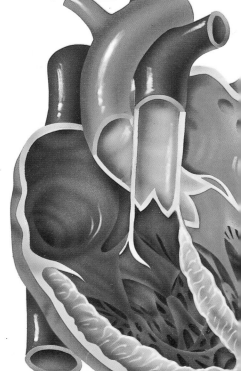

A heartbeat is really the "cardiac cycle" and has three phases:

1. First: Auricular systole and ventricular diastole. The auricle contracts and the blood passes from the auricle to the ventricle.

2. The ventricles are full; the tricuspid and mitral valves are closed.

3. Second: Ventricular systole. The ventricle contracts and increases the pressure. Blood comes out of the heart through the arteries.

4. Third: General diastole. The empty heart relaxes. The auricles and ventricles dilate so that the blood returns to the auricles.

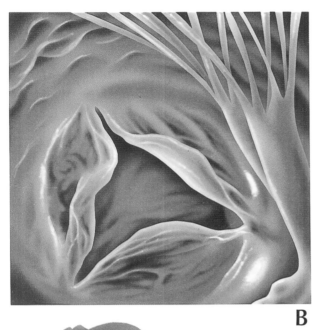

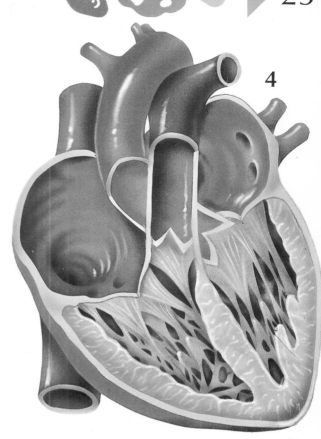

B

4

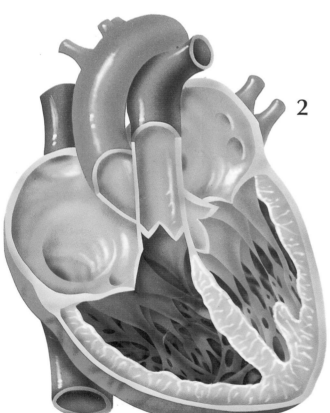

2

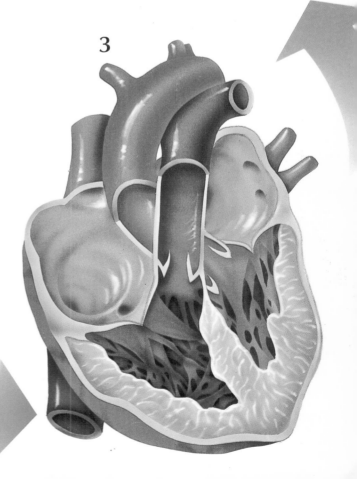

3

Blood leaves the right ventricle and flows toward the lungs, where it will be purified.

The heart pumps the blood to the lungs with less strength than it pumps blood through the aorta. This is why the right ventricle has four times less muscle than the left one.

When blood leaves the heart through the right ventricle, it is filled with carbon dioxide and has a blue color. It then travels through the pulmonary artery, which splits in two sections, each of which reaches one of the lungs. Then, each branch divides into smaller vessels to form a network of capillaries. In this network, the blood circulates slowly, which allows an exchange of gases with the lungs. When we breathe, air full of oxygen enters our lungs to the pulmonary alveoli.

Oxygenated blood reaches the left auricle through the pulmonary veins. It then goes to the left ventricle, and from there it is pumped to distribute oxygen to all the cells in the body.

Correct respiration is vital in getting oxygen to the pulmonary alveoli. The respiratory rhythm is also very important, since it is necessary to have enough time for carbon dioxide to be expelled during exhaling.

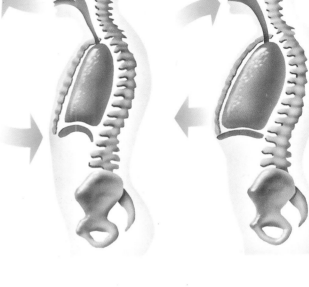

The route of the pulmonary circulation is much shorter than the systematic one. It only has to take the blood from the heart to the lungs and back to the heart.

Blood goes from the right auricle to the right ventricle of the heart and then comes out through the pulmonary arteries toward the lungs.

Pulmonary arteries split into smaller arteries to form the arterial capillaries that surround the pulmonary alveoli.

Then oxygen crosses the walls of the alveoli and reaches the blood capillaries that surround the alveoli like a net.

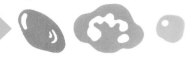

When air enters the lungs, oxygen reaches the blood capillaries.

The lungs have 300 million alveoli crossed by capillaries!

Logically, the exchange of gases is always from the areas where it is in larger amounts (higher pressure) to the ones where it is in a lesser amount.

The difference in pressure is actually between the blood capillaries and the pulmonary alveoli.

When we inhale, the amount of oxygen reaching the alveoli is greater than the amount of oxygen that exists in the capillaries. Therefore, part of the oxygen goes to the blood.

In the same way, there is a larger amount of carbon dioxide in the capillaries than there is in the alveoli, so the gas passes to the alveoli and then exits when we exhale.

In a day of normal respiration, one alveolus is filled and emptied more than 15,000 times.

1. The pulmonary alveoli are a part of the lung tissues and are shaped like a bunch of grapes surrounded by blood capillaries.

2. Oxygen crosses the membrane of the alveoli's walls and enters the red cells, where it attaches to hemoglobin molecules.

3. At the same time, carbon dioxide follows the same process, although in the opposite direction: going from the erythrocyte to the alveoli.

4. Carbon dioxide goes from the alveoli to the bronchial tubes and is finally expelled from the body during exhalation.

5. After passing through the alveoli, the capillaries that carry oxygenated erythrocyte group together to form the two pulmonary veins (one for each lung) that reach the left auricle of the heart.

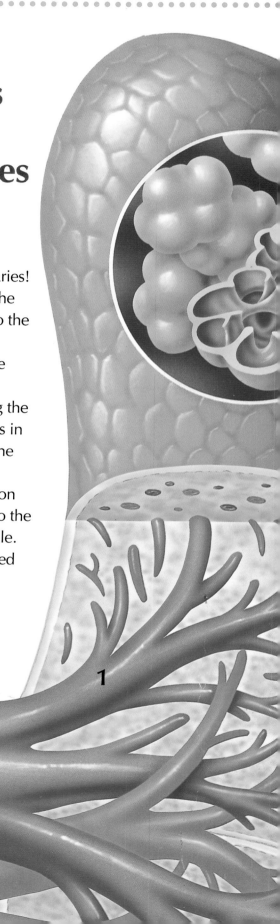

1

Erythrocytes must make an effort to pass through the capillaries that surround the alveoli. The air of the alveoli is at a distance of less than 0.000016 centimeters from the red cells and the exchange of gases is very quick.

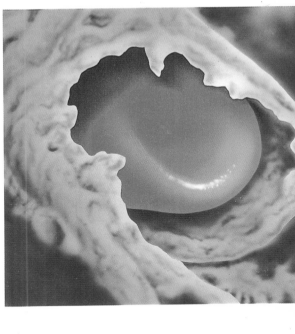

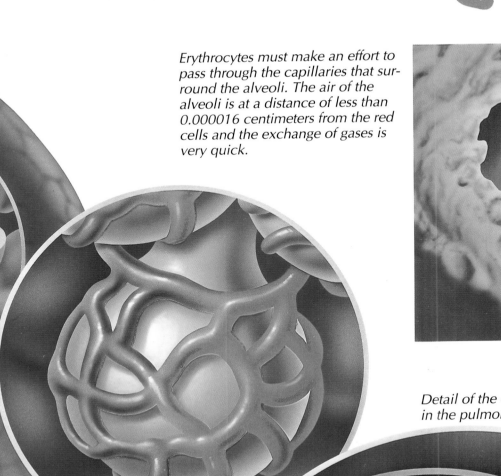

Detail of the exchange of gases in the pulmonary alveoli.

3

4

5

2

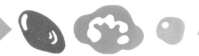

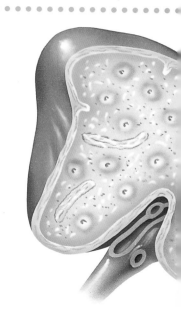

The blood carries substances that must be eliminated from the body through other organs.

To eliminate these toxic substances, the blood flows through different organs, such as the liver, spleen, and kidneys. Did you know that the liver is the most voluminous organ of the body? It weighs a little more than 3 pounds (1.5 kilograms). It is a fundamental organ since all the body's blood passes through it for purification and elimination of toxic substances. The liver filters the blood through the port vein, which branches out inside the liver into smaller veins that reach the surface of the hepatic lobes; the lobes are responsible for cleaning the blood.

The blood also passes through the kidneys to be cleaned. The spleen acts as the "cemetery" for the red cells. Every second it eliminates two million old red blood cells!

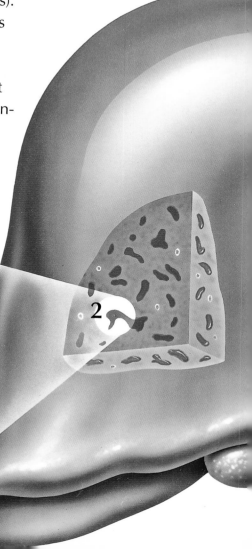

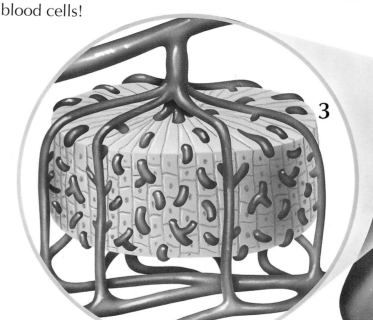

3

2

The spleen is a very special organ. In an emergency, it is able to release the blood inside to increase blood flow and oxygenation of the tissues.

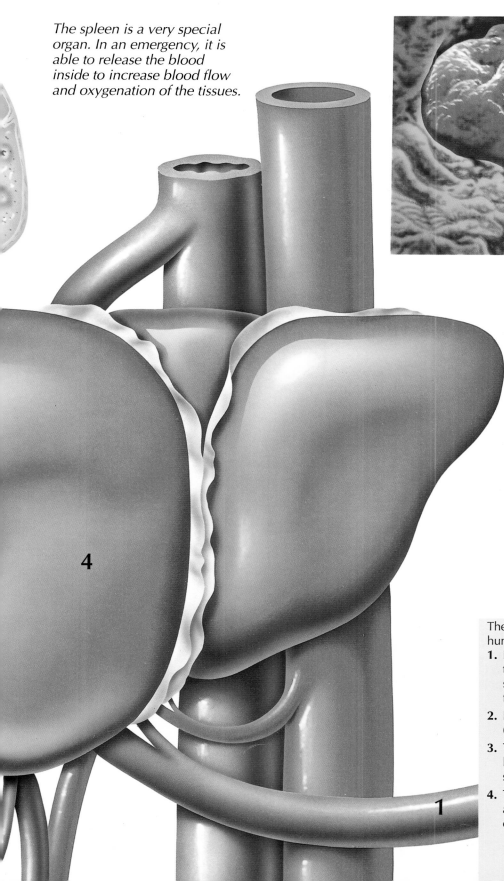

Each kidney contains more than one million nephrons, which work as blood-cleaning units. The blood passes through a complex group of capillaries called glomerals and the impurities are expelled in the urine.

The liver is the largest gland in the human body.

1. Blood enters the liver through the port vein and branches into smaller veins to reach the surface of the hepatic lobes.

2. In the lobes, hepatic cells (hepatocytes) filter the blood.

3. The blood is filtered and the liver retains the toxic substances that it has carried.

4. The liver, the bone marrow, and the spleen also filter blood clots in the circulatory system.

The lymphatic system is a second circulatory system in the human body.

The main function of this system is to collect the plasma that has gone from the capillaries to the tissues and carry it back to the blood. It prevents the flooding of the tissues.

The lymphatic system is made by a network of capillaries that form bigger vessels when they unite as in the vein system. Its walls are so thin that they allow the passage of proteins and large molecules that cannot be absorbed by blood capillaries.

The lymphatic system also has defense mechanisms. Along its vessels are enlarged areas called lymph nodes. Inside them, lymphocytes and macrophages mature and multiply (macrophages defend the body against potential infections). Also inside the lymph nodes are walls of membrane tissue that the lymph can cross. This membrane acts as a net for trapping bacteria and other foreign agents; lymphocytes then jump over and phagocytize them.

The human body has about one hundred lymph nodes, which are formed when several lymph vessels meet. Thanks to the lymphocytes they produce, they defend the body from attack by bacteria and microorganisms.

1

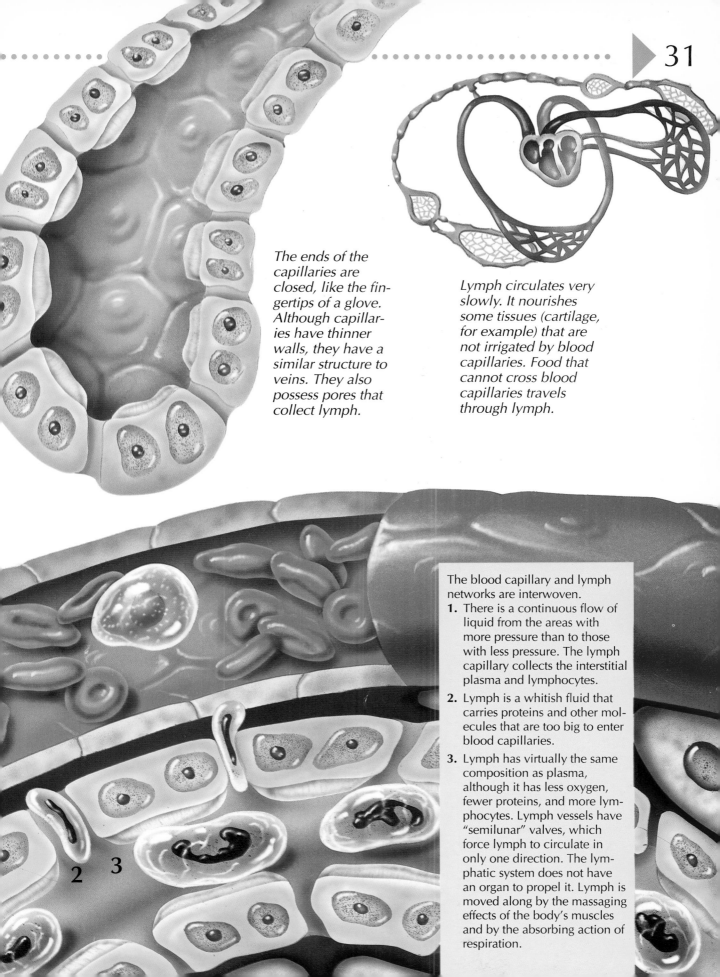

The ends of the capillaries are closed, like the fingertips of a glove. Although capillaries have thinner walls, they have a similar structure to veins. They also possess pores that collect lymph.

Lymph circulates very slowly. It nourishes some tissues (cartilage, for example) that are not irrigated by blood capillaries. Food that cannot cross blood capillaries travels through lymph.

2   3

The blood capillary and lymph networks are interwoven.

1. There is a continuous flow of liquid from the areas with more pressure than to those with less pressure. The lymph capillary collects the interstitial plasma and lymphocytes.

2. Lymph is a whitish fluid that carries proteins and other molecules that are too big to enter blood capillaries.

3. Lymph has virtually the same composition as plasma, although it has less oxygen, fewer proteins, and more lymphocytes. Lymph vessels have "semilunar" valves, which force lymph to circulate in only one direction. The lymphatic system does not have an organ to propel it. Lymph is moved along by the massaging effects of the body's muscles and by the absorbing action of respiration.

Glossary

Bacteria: Single-cell microorganisms that can be of many different types. Some are useful for agriculture, some cause diseases, some take part in fermentation and the putrefaction process, etc.

Cytoplasm: Substance that surrounds the nucleus of a cell. It has structures where most of the vital processes of the cell take place.

Diastole: Dilating movement whereby the heart is filled with the blood that reaches the auricles through the vena cava and pulmonary veins.

Fibrin: Support structure that produces a net called a "clot" in which the red blood cells are trapped, forming a lid that prevents the blood from escaping.

Hemoglobin: Protein in the red blood cells that is formed by four "hemo" (iron molecule) groups in which oxygen is transported.

Ion: An atom or a group of atoms or molecules that carries an electric charge as a result of having gained or lost electrons.

Molecule: A group of atoms that has all the properties of the substance it comes from.

Pigment: Coloring matter in a cell or tissue.

Plasma: Clear liquid in blood and in lymph where blood cells are present.

Pus: Yellowish liquid that is formed when leukocytes die fighting invading bacteria. It consists of dead leukocytes, dead and live bacteria, and cell waste swimming in the lymph.

Spleen: Large lymphatic vascular organ that is located in the abdominal cavity, under the diaphragm and on the left side. It filters the blood by removing the worn-out cells.

Systole: Contracting movement that expels blood from the heart.

Index